NAVIGATING NEW SKIES

A Pilot's Guide to Living Organ
Donation Campaigns

Written by an International Jet Pilot
/ Living Donor Kidney Recipient

Disclaimer:

The contents of this book, "Navigating New Skies: A Pilot's Guide to Living Organ Donation Campaigns," including all text, graphics, images, and other material contained herein, are for informational purposes only and do not constitute medical, legal, or other professional advice. The information is not intended to serve as a substitute for professional medical advice, diagnosis, or treatment. Always seek the advice of your physician, healthcare provider, or other qualified health providers with any questions you may have regarding a medical condition. Never disregard professional medical advice or delay seeking it because of something you have read in this book.

No part of this publication may be interpreted as a guarantee of specific outcomes. Individual results may vary, and there are numerous factors affecting the results of any organ donation campaign, many of which are beyond the control of the author and the services mentioned in this book.

The author has made every effort to ensure the accuracy of the information within this book was correct at the time of publication. The author does not assume and hereby disclaims any liability to any party for any loss, damage, or disruption caused by errors or omissions, whether such errors or omissions result from negligence, accident, or any other cause.

Readers should use their judgment and consult a variety of sources and professionals when making decisions affecting their health, well-being, and life choices. Additionally, readers are advised that the website and services mentioned in the book, TransplantPilot.com, come with no guarantees, and users should carefully review terms of service and policies before utilizing them.

This book is not a substitute for any legal or financial advice from professionals and all readers are encouraged to seek professional advice before making any decisions. The author disclaims any personal liability, both tangible and intangible, loss or risk incurred as a consequence of the use and application, either directly or indirectly, of any advice, information, or methods presented in this book.

All trademarks, service marks, trade names, trade dress, product names, and logos appearing in the book are the property of their respective owners. Any rights not expressly granted herein are reserved.

Remember, it's important that this disclaimer, or any legal text, is reviewed by a professional lawyer, especially one with experience in the publishing industry, to ensure you're fully protected and the disclaimer is comprehensive.

Acknowledgements

Before you delve into the pages that follow, I must express my deepest gratitude to those who have been the bedrock of my journey, the silent whispers of courage in my moments of doubt, and the raucous cheerleaders celebrating each small victory along my path.

To my incredible wife, whose unwavering love and strength have been my guiding lights through the darkest tunnels. Your belief in me, even when I struggled to believe in myself, has been nothing short of my salvation.

To my precious daughter, whose laughter is the melody I live to hear and whose future I strive to secure — you give me purpose beyond words and joy beyond measure.

To my loving mom, who first taught me resilience, who held my hand when I was weakest, and whose wisdom continues to fortify my spirit — you are my origin and my eternal home.

To my caring mother-in-law, whose kindness knows no bounds, and whose support has been as steadfast as a lighthouse in a storm — you are a blessing I never anticipated, but one I am eternally grateful for.

And most importantly, to Josh. Dear friend, my gratitude towards you transcends language. You came into my life as a beacon of hope and became the very pulse of my existence. Your selflessness is the reason I can embrace my wife and daughter each day. Because of your extraordinary gift, I have known the joy of watching sunrises and sunsets that I feared I would never see. You are not just my living donor; you are a savior in the truest sense. This book, my journey, and the additional time I've been given to cherish life's marvels — they are all testaments to your incredible humanity.

If it wasn't for your generosity, Josh, I wouldn't be living the great life I have been since my kidney transplant. You've not just given me a second chance at life; you've redefined the very essence of my existence.

So, with a heart brimming with gratitude, I dedicate this work to all of you. You are the heroes of my story — the one that I am privileged to continue writing each day, thanks to you.

With love and endless gratitude,

Sebastian

Table of Contents

Chapter 1:

Lift-Off: A Pilot's Journey to Second Chances

Part 1: The Uninvited Turbulence

My life revolved around the powerful hum of jet engines, the endless horizon stretching out from the cockpit, and the unique thrill that came with controlling a Gulfstream. A corporate pilot's life might look glamorous from the outside—flying CEOs and executives worldwide, brushing shoulders with power, and frequently dotting the globe's skies. Yet, it's a life stitched together by an unspoken code of honor, precision, and immense responsibility.

That fateful Sunday was cloaked in deception—a day of leisure, an afternoon with friends, the air echoing with the crack of baseball bats and fans' roars at a Phillies game. But as I bit into a dollar hot dog, laughter mingling with chatter, an unrelenting back pain gnawed at my focus, an ominous whisper that this was just the beginning of a new, unwelcome chapter.

Part 2: Navigating the Genetic Storm

I was no stranger to PKD. It ran in the family, a silent specter haunting our lineage. My mom had been its victim, and her journey was nothing short of heroic. Memories of hospital visits, doctors' grim expressions, and my stepdad's incredible act of love and donation were all embedded in my childhood narrative.

So, when my back pain culminated in a diagnosis that echoed my past, it wasn't shock that gripped me—it was an icy realization. The following days were a blur of hospital corridors, the sterile smell of medical reports, and probing questions that seemed to strip my dreams layer by layer. After an agonizing two-month hiatus filled with more medical exams than I could count, the skies welcomed me again—but this time, the clouds were tinged with the shadow of PKD.

Part 3: Eleven Years in the Eye of the Storm

For eleven years, I flew. Above the clouds, PKD was just a distant thunderstorm. Yet, on the ground, it was my ever-present shadow. Every six months, like clockwork, the FAA medicals loomed. Each was an ordeal, a biannual gamble with my destiny. Would I fly again, or would this be the end? The stress was a relentless hum in the background of my life, always there, always waiting.

But life... life doesn't pause for fear. My daughter's laughter was my daily reprieve, her wide-eyed wonder a reminder that some things were bigger than my fears. And my wife—my rock, my guiding star—her strength was my sanctuary.

We searched for a Plan B, a safety net, something that whispered security. I pored over opportunities, but nothing fit. Nothing quelled the storm that brewed on our horizon.

Part 4: Grounded, But Not Defeated

The day my wings were clipped was unremarkable to the world. No thunder, no lightning—just a simple, crushing sentence: "Your kidney function is too low." But surrender was never in my flight plan. We took the fight head-on, charting unknown territories of the human spirit.

Night after night, when the world faded to silence, I spoke to my daughter through the camera lens, encapsulating life lessons, love, laughter—creating a vault of memories she could revisit.

Part 5: Before the Storm—A Father's Love

The eve of my surgery wasn't marked by panic; it was quieter, reflective, almost solemn. Surrounded by the sterile white walls of my hospital room, my wife's hand found mine—a silent pact. We didn't need words; our hearts spoke volumes. That night, I wasn't a pilot, a patient, or a warrior—I was a father, a husband, terrified of the unspoken "what-ifs."

Part 6: The Journey Envisioned

This book isn't a mere recount of events. It's a lighthouse for souls lost in the tempest, proof that even in our darkest moments, we aren't alone. It's a manual for braving personal storms, a tale of triumph, fear, love, and resilience. Ahead, there will be turbulence, moments of despair, and soaring heights. But together, we'll navigate, because hope guides us, love uplifts us, and courage propels us forward. Strap in—it's time to take off.

Chapter 2:

Pre-flight Check: Understanding Organ Donation

Part 1: The Basics of Organ Donation

Stepping into the world of organ donation was like being handed the controls of a jet with no flight training. But just like flying, the more you understand, the less daunting it becomes. So, let's break it down.

We've got two types of organ donation: living and deceased. Living donors can donate a kidney or a part of the liver, lung, intestine, or pancreas. And did you know? A kidney from a living donor can last 15–20 years. That's a lot of extra sunrises, folks. Deceased donors can give all organs, tissues, and even eyes.

But there are myths out there muddying the waters. Age is a big one. Many think there's an age limit, but the truth is, there's no expiry date on being a hero. Eligibility is determined by medical criteria at the time of death, not the candles on your birthday cake. And let's talk living donation. Some people aren't aware they can donate an organ while they're still breathing and enjoy a healthy life afterward. We need to bust these myths wide open because, with more accurate information, more lives can be saved.

Part 2: The Urgency

Ready for some turbulence? Hold on to your hats. As of 2022, there were 88,901 people just in the U.S. waiting on a life-saving kidney. But it doesn't stop there. Add in the thousands waiting for livers, hearts, and other organs, and you've got yourself an urgent crisis. Global organ transplantations hit over 144,000 in 2021, but it's still not enough to meet the demand.

Every day, hopeful individuals are watching sunsets, wondering if they'll get the call. And it's not just numbers on a page; these are real people with families, dreams, and stories left to write. It's up to us to spread awareness and get more folks registered as donors. It's not just a kind gesture; it's a matter of life.

Part 3: The Living Donation

Living donation? It's like giving someone a boarding pass for an extended, joy-filled journey. But it's not without its trials. Donors undergo thorough evaluations and recovery, which isn't a walk in the park. But the consensus? "It's worth it." With living donation, we're not just talking about saving lives; we're talking about enriching them, too.

Part 4: Navigating Legal and Ethical Skies

The legal landscape here is as crucial as the medical one. You can't sell organs; that's a big no-no worldwide. The National Organ Transplant Act ensures the U.S. keeps a level playing field, where organs go to those in dire need, not the highest bidder. It's about fairness, ethics, and giving each person in need a fighting chance.

Part 5: The Emotional and Psychological Runway

This journey is a whirlwind of emotions, from the fear of the unknown to the joy of a second chance. It's vital to acknowledge this and know that it's okay to seek help. Organizations like OneLegacy offer grief support, and the American Liver Foundation has a hotline for those with concerns or questions. And let's not forget the importance of communication. Professionals, like those at The Organ Donation and Transplantation Alliance, are dedicated to making these tough conversations easier and more informed.

Remember, whether you're a donor, a recipient, or a supportive loved one, you're never flying solo on this journey.

Chapter 3:

Gaining Altitude: Navigating the Emotional Journey

Part 1: Turbulence Ahead: Recognizing the Emotional Challenges

Buckle up, friends. This journey through the skies of organ donation isn't just about the physical. Indeed, it's an emotional rollercoaster, with peaks of hope and valleys of despair. It's normal to feel a storm of emotions — fear, anxiety, even guilt, or anger. These feelings aren't signposts to weakness, but markers of our shared humanity. Remember, acknowledging our emotions is the first step to managing them, like spotting a storm on the horizon and adjusting your flight path accordingly.

Part 2: The Support Crew: Finding Your Emotional Support System

No pilot flies solo through a storm, and neither should you. Your support crew — family, friends, counselors, spiritual leaders, or support groups — is crucial. They're the co-pilots, air traffic controllers, and ground crew in your journey, helping navigate the rough patches. And don't underestimate the power of connecting with others in the same airspace. Sharing experiences with those who truly understand can be as comforting as a beacon in the night sky.

Part 3: In-Flight Mechanics: Strategies for Emotional Well-being

Maintaining emotional equilibrium on this flight is key, and it's more proactive than you'd think. Develop coping strategies that work for you, whether that's mindfulness, meditation, exercise, journaling, or a hobby that keeps your spirits soaring. These are your in-flight mechanics, crucial for the journey's smooth sailing. Remember, a little turbulence is normal, but you've got the tools to ride it out.

Part 4: The Compass Within: Trusting Your Decision-Making

When you're cruising at altitude, doubts can cloud your judgment like fog over a runway. Am I making the right choice? What are the risks? What if, what if, what if? Trust your compass within. You've gathered information, consulted with experts, weighed the pros and cons, and listened to your gut. Trusting yourself is the instrument panel of decision-making; it helps navigate through the clouds of uncertainty.

Part 5: Safe Landing: Preparing for Post-Donation Life

The journey doesn't end with the act of donating or receiving; oh no, it's just a new beginning. Prepare for the changes. Plan for the recovery. Embrace the new normal. It might involve some readjustments and accommodations, but what's a landing without a bit of braking, right? And give yourself a pat on the back; whether you're giving or receiving, you've embarked on one of the most profound journeys of the human experience.

Remember, this flight path isn't set in stone. It winds and changes, with bright skies and stormy weather. But with courage, support, and a bit of navigational know-how, we'll reach a destination worth every bit of the journey. Safe flying, my friends.

Chapter 4:

Plotting the Course: Personalized Marketing Strategies

Before we dive into the specifics of crafting your personalized marketing strategy, it's essential to understand why this step is so crucial. Searching for an organ isn't just a wait; it's a proactive journey. In today's digital age, merely hoping for the best isn't enough. You need to seize control of your narrative and actively reach out, and that's where a well-thought-out marketing plan comes into play.

A marketing plan is your roadmap. It's an organized framework that gives your search direction, visibility, and structure. Why is this so important? Here are a few reasons:

Visibility: There are countless voices in the online and offline world. A marketing plan helps you stand out, be heard, and be remembered. It's about making sure your story reaches the eyes and ears it needs to, whether that's potential donors, supporters, or organizations that can help.

Control: Your story is deeply personal, and it should be told your way. A marketing plan allows you to control the narrative, ensuring that your journey is portrayed authentically and that your needs and goals are clearly communicated.

Mobilization: You're not just building awareness; you're rallying support. A good marketing plan turns passive listeners into active participants. They're not just sympathizing; they're signing up, spreading the word, and actively contributing to your search.

Efficiency: Time is of the essence, and resources can be limited. A marketing plan ensures that your efforts are strategic, targeted, and efficient. It's about making the most significant impact with what you have, without burning out or getting lost in the noise.

Hope: This journey is emotional, and it can feel overwhelming. A marketing plan is a commitment to yourself and your supporters. It's a tangible, proactive step forward. It says, "I'm not giving up. I have a plan, and I'm going to fight." That's powerful.

In the search for an organ, a marketing plan is more than a strategy; it's a lifeline. It connects you with the people who can turn your hope into a reality. It's not a guarantee of success, but it significantly increases your chances. It's about taking your hope into your own hands and giving it a voice—a voice that can reach across the street or across the globe.

Now, let's delve into how exactly you can create this lifeline.

Part 1: The Need for a Personalized Plan - Crafting Your Story

Summary:

In this initial phase, you're going to delve deep into your own journey. This is where your campaign begins — with a story that's uniquely yours. You'll need to articulate your experiences, your struggles, and your hopes in a way that others not only understand but also emotionally connect with. This personal narrative is crucial because it's not just your story; it becomes your campaign's identity.

Action Steps:

- Draft Your Story: Spend time reflecting on your journey. What were the pivotal moments? How did they change you? Write it down in a narrative style, highlighting moments of struggle, hope, and resilience.

- Collect Multimedia Content: Photos, videos, and voice notes add a multi-dimensional aspect to your story. Collect content from different phases of your journey, including images or videos from hospital visits, treatment sessions, daily life, and special events that illustrate your experience.

- Establish Clear Objectives: What exactly do you hope to achieve with your campaign? Is it finding a donor, raising funds for medical expenses, or perhaps both? Having precise, measurable goals will give your campaign a sense of purpose and direction.

Part 2: Understanding Your Audience - The Heart of Your Community

Summary:

Now, it's time to understand who you're speaking to. Every successful campaign knows its audience — their preferences, their hangouts, their hearts. You're not just broadcasting a message; you're building relationships with a community ready to listen, help, and spread the word.

Action Steps:

- Audience Research: Conduct surveys or have conversations with potential audience groups to understand their perspectives, challenges, and motivations. Consider age, location, cultural background, and experiences with organ donation or health challenges.

- Customize Communication Strategies: Different demographics have unique communication preferences. Younger audiences might prefer social media, while older individuals may engage more with emails or community newsletters. Plan your communication methods accordingly.

- Develop Engagement Initiatives: Plan for live Q&A sessions, create interactive posts, or host virtual community gatherings. The aim is to foster a two-way relationship that makes your audience feel valued and involved.

Part 3: Outlining Your Flight Plan - Developing a Step-by-Step Campaign

Summary:

A journey of a thousand miles begins with a single step — and a well-thought-out plan. What are the milestones of your campaign? What content will you share and when? A structured approach lets you navigate your path systematically and allows your audience to follow along and be part of your journey.

Action Steps:

- Construct a Detailed Timeline: Break down your campaign into phases. What do you plan to achieve during each of these stages? Include specific tasks, like launching a website, starting a social media challenge, or hosting a fundraising event, and assign deadlines.

- Integrate "Done for You" Services: Not everyone has the time or expertise to manage a full-scale marketing campaign. This is where transplantpilot.com comes in. Our range of services can be tailored to suit your needs, whether it's content creation, community management, event planning, or complete campaign management. Assess which areas you need the most support in and let professionals handle them for you. This not only elevates the quality of your campaign but also allows you to focus on your well-being and family.

- Coordinate Professional Services: If you're considering "done for you" services, now's the time to integrate them into your plan. Determine which aspects of your campaign you need assistance with, such as graphic design, website management, or public relations, and schedule these services.

Part 4: Branding Your Journey - Making Your Mark

Summary:

Your brand is more than a logo; it's an identity. It's what people will recognize, relate to, and remember. A consistent, personalized brand makes your campaign more professional and memorable. It's not just about visibility; it's about making a lasting impression.

Action Steps:

- Design Your Brand Identity: This goes beyond just a logo. What colors, fonts, and imagery will represent your journey? Ensure they resonate with your story's emotions. Your tagline should be concise, memorable, and impactful.

- Implement Brand Consistency: Use your brand elements across all materials. From your social media pages to your fundraising materials, consistency enhances recognition and trust.

- Create Symbolic Merchandise: Think of items that supporters would be proud to wear or display. Whether it's T-shirts with your campaign logo or custom bracelets, choose merchandise that carries your message effectively.

Part 5: Tools for Navigation - Resources, Tools, and Services for Your Unique Journey

Summary:

The digital age offers a plethora of tools to streamline your campaign, from content creation to audience engagement. Understanding and utilizing these tools can maximize your efficiency and reach. Moreover, continual learning is crucial — stay updated with the latest trends and technologies to keep your campaign fresh and engaging.

Action Steps:

- Assemble Your Digital Toolbox: Identify software and platforms that will aid in content creation, social media management, fundraising, and community engagement. Set these up early to streamline your processes.

- Explore Comprehensive Solutions at transplantpilot.com: While assembling your toolbox, don't forget to explore the extensive resources and "done for you" services available at transplantpilot.com. From personalized marketing strategies to handling logistical complexities, these professional services are designed to lighten your load and enhance your campaign's effectiveness. Schedule a consultation to discuss your needs and discover how we can collaborate to navigate your journey successfully.

- Engage Expert Services: Consider which aspects of your campaign could benefit from professional touch—graphic design, copywriting, or even legal advice. Research and reach out to experts or agencies who align with your mission.

Your path through this challenging time doesn't have to be a solitary journey. There are numerous resources and professional services designed to help guide you through. Your story is waiting to be told, and we at transplantpilot.com are here to help amplify your voice. Let's embark on this journey together!

Fly Healthy!

Chapter 5:

Takeoff: Launching Your Campaign

Introductory Summary:

In this chapter, you'll be guided through the critical phase of bringing your campaign to life. We'll delve into the meticulous preparation, the excitement of the launch, and the ongoing effort to maintain momentum. This isn't just about what you need to do; it's also about understanding where expert services, available at TransplantPilot.com, can elevate your campaign. It's about ensuring that your message doesn't just reach people, but moves them.

Part 1: Pre-launch Checklist - Ensuring a Smooth Takeoff

Summary:

Before you unveil your campaign to the world, a comprehensive pre-launch check is essential. This involves not just a review of your content, but an affirmation that your campaign's heart and soul — your story — is communicated effectively. For areas outside your expertise, professional services are available at TransplantPilot.com to ensure no stone is left unturned.

Action Steps:

In-depth Narrative Review: Immerse yourself in your story once more. Does it convey the emotions and the urgency authentically? Are your mission and call-to-action clear? TransplantPilot.com offers storytelling assistance, perfect for capturing the essence of your journey compellingly.

Comprehensive Technical Trial Run: Ensure all technical aspects, from website functionality to mobile responsiveness, are flawless. Technical issues should not hamper your story's reach. For technical support, TransplantPilot.com has you covered.

Support Crew Briefing: Every team member should be clear on their roles and the campaign's core message. If team coordination is daunting, consider professional support orchestration from TransplantPilot.com.

Resource Audit: Double-check your educational materials and FAQ sections. Clarity and compassion are key in these resources. Professional content review and creation are available at TransplantPilot.com.

Part 2: The Launch - Your Story Takes Flight

Summary:

This is the moment your campaign truly begins. It's more than pressing "Go Live"; it's about actively engaging with your initial audience, setting the tone, and closely monitoring the response to adapt quickly. Remember, you're not alone in this; TransplantPilot.com's services are designed to help you manage this process efficiently.

Action Steps:

Initial Engagement: Respond promptly and personally to initial feedback and engagement. Your first responders will be your strongest advocates. For those needing assistance with community management, TransplantPilot.com provides engagement services.

Monitoring Performance: Use analytics to track your campaign's reach and engagement. Understand what's working and what needs adjustment. If data analysis isn't your strength, TransplantPilot.com offers performance monitoring services.

Adapt and Modify: Be ready to tweak your message or approach based on audience response. Flexibility could make the difference between fizzling interest and growing momentum. For strategy adaptation, turn to the experts at TransplantPilot.com.

Part 3: Maintaining Altitude - Keeping the Momentum Going

Summary:

A successful campaign doesn't end after the launch; maintaining momentum is key. This involves consistent engagement, refreshing your content, and keeping your audience invested in your journey. It's also recognizing when to leverage external expertise from resources like TransplantPilot.com to keep your campaign soaring.

Action Steps:

Regular Updates: Keep your audience involved with consistent, meaningful updates. They're invested in your journey; don't let them feel forgotten. If creating ongoing content is overwhelming, TransplantPilot.com offers content creation services.

Audience Engagement: Continue building relationships with your audience. Ask for their stories, their advice, their hopes. If managing this continuous engagement is daunting, community management services are available at TransplantPilot.com.

Refresh and Revitalize: Periodically inject new life into your campaign with fresh content, new stories, or exciting announcements. For those struggling with creative strategies, TransplantPilot.com provides campaign revitalization services.

Part 4: Navigation and Adjustment - When to Change Course

Sumary:

No journey is without turbulence. There will be moments when strategies need to be reassessed and changes made. This part focuses on understanding the signs that it's time to change course and how to do it adeptly, with a reminder that professional guidance is available at TransplantPilot.com to help navigate these moments.

Action Steps:

Performance Assessment: Regularly review campaign analytics to gauge what's effective and what's not. If you're uncertain how to interpret the data or take the next steps, TransplantPilot.com offers consulting services.

Feedback Incorporation: Actively seek out and thoughtfully consider audience feedback. Sometimes, the most insightful directions come from those following your journey. If you need assistance in collecting or utilizing feedback, turn to TransplantPilot.com.

Strategic Pivoting: Don't be afraid to change strategies or try new approaches. Innovation keeps your campaign fresh and engaging. If you're unsure about the next best step, strategic planning services are available at TransplantPilot.com.

Chapter 6:

The Journey Ahead

Summary:

In this final chapter, we reflect on the journey we've embarked on together. We'll recap the key strategies discussed, ponder the emotional journey ahead, and consider the next steps as you bring your campaign to life. Remember, the road may be long, but you're not walking it alone — resources like TransplantPilot.com are here to help you navigate the path forward.

Part 1. Recap of Key Strategies:

In the preceding chapters, we delved deep into the intricacies of organizing a campaign, from emotional preparedness to mobilizing support, from personalized marketing strategies to funding. It's essential to remember the core tenets of authenticity, detailed planning, and consistent communication in your campaign. The personalized approach isn't just a tactic; it's a reflection of your unique journey, resonating with those who are ready to support you.

Part 2. Emotional Considerations:

This journey is laden with emotions. It's normal to experience highs and lows, hope and despair. Surround yourself with a support system—friends, family, therapists, or support groups. Remember, taking care of your mental health is as crucial as the physical aspects of this journey. Allow yourself to feel, understand that setbacks are not the end, and celebrate every small victory along the way.

Part 3. Planning Your Next Steps:

What's next is putting this plan into action. Start with small, manageable steps. Maybe that's setting up a meeting with your inner circle to discuss strategies, or perhaps it's reaching out to a professional service to kickstart your campaign. Keep the momentum going, and remember, consistency is key. Regularly revisit your plan, adjust as necessary, and remember, each step forward is a step toward your goal.

Part 4. Additional Resources:

Beyond this book, there are numerous resources at your disposal. Online platforms, community groups, and healthcare providers can offer invaluable support. Continuously educate yourself about new strategies and technologies emerging in the field of campaign marketing and funding. Knowledge is not just power; it's the fuel for your journey.

Part 5. Closing Thoughts and Gratitude:

As we wrap up this guide, I want to leave you with a message of hope and gratitude. Hope for the journey ahead, and gratitude for your courage to embark on this path. Remember, your story is powerful, your life is valuable, and your journey is worth every effort.

Part 6. Your Companion on This Journey — TransplantPilot.com:

You're not alone on this journey. If you're feeling overwhelmed or in need of specialized help, remember that TransplantPilot.com offers a range of 'done for you' services. From creating personalized marketing plans to executing detailed campaign strategies, professional assistance is just a click away. Utilizing these services can give your campaign the professional touch it needs, allowing you to focus on your well-being.

Part 7. Invitation for Ongoing Dialogue:

This book is just the beginning of an ongoing conversation. I encourage you to reach out with your stories, questions, and feedback. Share your successes and your setbacks. Not only does this help improve future editions of this guide, but it also strengthens the community we're building together. Your journey could be the inspiration someone else needs to begin theirs.

Final Conclusion and Thank You:

As we close the pages of this guide, it's not an end but a beginning — the start of your unique journey. The road ahead will have its shares of ups and downs, but every step forward is a victory. It's a path we now walk together, in solidarity and hope.

I want to extend my deepest gratitude to you, the reader. Thank you for letting me be a part of your journey, for embracing the strategies, and for your commitment to forging ahead even when times get tough. Your strength inspires, and your journey matters — not just to you, but to your loved ones and the broader community rallying behind you.

As you embark on this new chapter, remember that you carry with you the wisdom, the plans, and the heartfelt energy from all the chapters before this. You are equipped, you are not alone, and you are valued. Keep the faith, stay the course, and never hesitate to reach out for help when you need it. Your story is waiting to unfold, and the world is ready to cheer you on.

Thank you for bringing me along on your journey. Here's to hope, to health, and to the incredible journey ahead.

Fly healthy!

Sebastian

Pilot & Living Donor Kidney Recipient

www.transplantpilot.com